100 Hints:
How To Live To A Healthy 100

*Secrets from those who've reached 100,
or soon will!*

By Russ L. Potter, II

How To Live To A Healthy 100
Secrets from those who've made it, or are well on their way!
ISBN 1-57757-002-2

Copyright ©1996 by The Concerned Group, Inc.
P.O. Box 1000
Siloam Springs, Arkansas 72761

Published by **Trade Life Books, Inc.**
P.O. Box 55325
Tulsa, Oklahoma 74155

Dedication

For his consistent example and inspiration over the years, this book is lovingly dedicated to my father, Russell L. Potter, Sr. — 93 years old and still taking cold showers!

Special Thanks

The following people generously contributed their time, energy and talents in the development of this edition. Sincere appreciation is extended to the following people: Judy Adkins, Cindy Blount, Sheila Blount, Felicia Graham, Julie Hill, Jeanne Jensen, Sara Jensen, Rich LaVere, Bill Morelan, Sheri Morelan, Gordon Rich, Riki Stamps, Lou Stewart, and Paula Taylor. And, most of all, thanks to the wonderful people who shared their wisdom in the following pages!

Introduction

When we're young, life seems like an open-ended lease. It's there for as long as we choose to live it! We can stay up all night, eat and drink whatever our taste buds call for, and "exercise" is simply the natural result of dashing on to our next destination!

But life doesn't stay that way. Soon, we can't quite drive all night, certain foods no longer agree with us and exercise is something we mostly just "think" about!

Recently, when my Aunt Faith passed up seconds on her birthday cake, I asked her for any other "health wisdom" she might have stored up on her way to 103!

Her sharp wit and rapid replies confirmed the things my dad had been telling me for years — advice that made even more sense now that I had reached half-a-hundred!

I've long wished to collect and publish the remarkable insights I've gained from those people who have lived long, abundant and healthy lives. So, I continued to ask others in their 80's, 90's & 100's what thoughts they might have to share.

The following pages contain amazing secrets and helpful hints from those who have "lived with vitality" beyond the "average." Perhaps, from this collage of wisdom, you too will discover the incentives to reconsider and then transform your life for good!

Yours for longer, healthier living!

Russ Potter

Russ L. Potter, II

Hobbies & Interests

Hint #1

"Keep doing the things you like as long as you're able."

Gladyce Kroll
August 9, 1911
Soldier, Iowa

"I like to do a lot of everything," says Gladyce. "Stay active. Don't waste time thinking about growing old!" Gladyce played basketball for many years, and until recently played golf three times a week.

Hint #2

"Don't be afraid to get your hands dirty."

Thelma Cogswell
February 12, 1911
Washington, D.C.

Thelma has been an avid gardener since she was old enough to hold a garden trowel. She is a member of "Friendship Through Flowers," and enjoys sharing her love for flowers with others.

Hint #3

***"You're never too old for dolls or pets —
they're great company."***

Ruth Blow
December 23, 1911
Kensington, Pennsylvania

Ruth has been a widow for over a decade, but she never feels lonely because she always has her pet poodle, Yanni, by her side. Her home is filled with an extensive doll collection which she has accumulated over most of her life.

Hint #4

"Don't be afraid to try new things!"

M. Ruth Burch
August 2, 1916
Blaine, Michigan

Over the years, Ruth has done everything from building her own cabinets to creating exquisite oil paintings. She even drew up the architectural plans for her home. Ruth now spends her mornings in the kitchen cooking for her numerous grandchildren, great-grandchildren, and members of her extended family.

Hint #5

"Relax and enjoy the scenery.
Visit beautiful places if you can."

Marjorie Brown
February 2, 1912
Fletcher, North Carolina

Marjorie has visited many beautiful places, including Alaska and Hawaii. She says traveling always gives her something to look forward to, and she finds it "restful."

Hint #6

"Read a lot. It continually broadens your horizons."

Ruth Ingram
June 15, 1911
Lilesville, North Carolina

Ruth, who taught school for 42 years, didn't attend formal school herself until the sixth grade. She started reading at four years old, "and I've never stopped," she says. Just recently, she finished reading *My American Journey*, a 644-page book by General Colin Powell.

Hint #7

"Study God's Word and believe it to be true."

Allie Belle Root
October 29, 1902
Rogers, Arkansas

Allie was born in her grandparent's home. After graduation, she taught school for nearly 35 years. "I never missed a single day of classes," she says. "And in all that time I was never late once."

Hint #8

*"Have good friends. It's made
a difference in my life."*

Fern Willett
April 1, 1909
Minneapolis, Minnesota

Fern believes in having an active social life. She is still best friends
with her college roommate from the class of 1927.

Hint #9

*"Keep a pet. They're kind
and faithful companions."*

Clive Possinger
February 9, 1907
Tobyhanna, Pennsylvania

Clive's dog "Mimi" has been his faithful companion for over nine years. He has had a variety of pets through the years including dogs, birds, a fox, and even a skunk. "Skunks are a lot like kittens," he grins.

Hint #10

*"Balance your activities —
mental and physical."*

Merywn Bridenstine
May 1, 1902
Iowa City, Iowa

Although Merywn made his living as a business administration professor and college dean, he always kept busy around the house. He says, "Over the years I've painted, built an addition, done concrete work, re-shingled the roof — and kept busy in the garden too!"

Hint #11

"Stay active by being a good listener."

Beulah Graham
April 18, 1910
Long Point, Illinois

Over the years, Beulah has been a volunteer for many church and civic organizations. She is "grandma" to hundreds of people, including many at Turning Point — a shelter for battered women and children.

Hint #12

"Spend your days working hard in the fresh air."

Ervin Langley
March 13, 1907
St. Paul, Arkansas

Ervin has always worked outdoors — first on apple ranches in Washington state, and later doing utility work in northeast Oklahoma. "I chose good ancestors, too," he grins. His mother was one of 13 children, most of whom lived well into their 90s.

Hint #13

"Volunteer your time and talents to help others."

Harry Winton
April 7, 1920
Sayre, Pennsylvania

Harry is an active volunteer for a senior citizen program, delivering 18 meals a day to "the elderly," and calling shut-ins to check on their physical condition. "As much as people appreciate what we do," says Harry, "I think we volunteers get the biggest blessing!"

Hint #14

"Never sit still; always stay busy!"

Emma Points
April 15, 1906
Baxter Springs, Kansas

Emma is a firm believer in the old saying, "When you rest, you rust." She has been a housewife most of her life and today she keeps busy sewing together handmade quilts.

Hint #15

"Just stay active."

Effie Lee Elkins
July 14, 1897
Huntsville, Arkansas

Effie has been going strong all her life. In addition to raising seven children, she worked as a cook in a cafe, and later in a cannery. "I bowled until I was 89," says Effie, "and I've fished all my life."

Hint #16

"Play a lot of golf...and laugh a lot!"

Ruby Graham
June 7, 1910
Green Camp, Ohio

Ruby has won several golf tournaments in Ohio and Florida. Both of her parents died when she was only three years old. She recommends, "Don't spend too much time crying over things you can't help!"

Hint #17

***"Mow your yard regularly...
it clears the mind!"***

Lettieteen Blount
February 12, 1915
French Settlement, Louisiana

Lettieteen hasn't let the years interfere with her love of nature. She still has one of the best-kept yards in town. She also tries to take time each day, "just to watch the flowers grow."

Hint #18

"Keep yourself busy!"

Ethel Elder
September 12, 1910
Madison County, Arkansas

Ethel has been active all her life. In addition to helping her husband on the farm, Ethel raised six children — doing all the family laundry on a washboard! Today, if she's not out working in her vegetable garden, she's usually sewing on one of her hand-made quilts.

Hint #19

*"Plant lots of flowers.
Flowers keep you young."*

Mary Strickland
December 29, 1899
Marion, Ohio

Mary says having a green thumb has kept her busy all her life. "We always had a huge garden and lived off the land," she says. Mary still enjoys having lots of flowers around.

Hint #20

"Travel, travel, travel."

Leona Turner
October 13, 1903
Chanute, Kansas

Leona has visited all 50 states and Canada and Mexico! She says she's always had the "travel bug." She enjoys mapping out trips with a friend and traveling mostly by car.

Hint #21

"Keep your mind active, the rest will follow."

Marie Blaha
August 30, 1898
Cleveland, Ohio

Marie worked as a sales clerk/bookkeeper for the famous Frederick's of Hollywood. She was nearly 80 before she stopped working full-time. "I still like to keep busy," she says, "even though I've had to slow down a little bit."

Hint #22

"Always take time for simple pleasures."

Emma Porter
April 15, 1900
Lampasas, Texas

Emma grew up on a cotton farm in Texas. "We always worked hard, but had fun anyway," she laughs. "I still remember stopping every so often to sing together. . .but we didn't stop for long!" At age 96, she raised almost $300 walking in the "Miles for Meals" fund-raiser.

Hint #23

"Always be willing to share."

Helen Stamper
October 19, 1910
Augusta, Georgia

Helen, the eldest of five children, has always enjoyed "doin' for others." She spends most of her time collecting small gifts, pretty cards, and humorous quotes to give to her friends and neighbors.

Hint #24

"Study your Bible every day."

Geneva Baskin
October 28, 1907
Union County, North Carolina

Geneva didn't have any sisters, but was always very close to her cousin, Novella. They shared grief together when their husbands died, but they also shared their abiding faith.

Hint #25

"Take time to watch a baseball game."

Milton Ewald
May 12, 1917
Haven, Wisconsin

Milton believes you must stay physically active to remain healthy — he's an avid bicycle rider. But he also believes that it can be therapeutic to watch young people perform at sporting events.

Hint #26

"For a long life, listen to your parents. That's Biblical!"

Mabel Cherry
October 2, 1902
Gravette, Arkansas

Mabel Cherry says she's always tried to follow what her parents taught her. She still enjoys reminders of the past — like listening to the "old time gospel songs" and meeting up with old acquaintances.

Nutrition & Exercise

Hint #27

"Get exercise every day doing something you like."

Guy Harris
August 16, 1910
Wellston, Oklahoma

Guy retired over twenty years ago, but he still enjoys working in his son-in-law's racing stables. As part of his "chores," he feeds and waters the horses twice each day — rain or shine!

Hint #28

"Work hard and eat lots of fresh vegetables."

Jeffery Blount, Sr.
November 6, 1912
Denham Springs, Louisiana

Jeffery has grown a garden every summer for over 60 years! Each fall he fills his freezer, and then shares the rest of his harvest with neighbors. He also keeps a few goats "just for the fun of it."

Hint #29

"Don't drink anything cold, and get regular exercise."

Marguerita Wood
September 14, 1907
Kiowa County, Oklahoma Territory

Marguerita drinks several glasses of warm water each day, and relies on her exercise bike to stay in shape. "I'm glad they don't charge by the mile," she laughs. "The meter broke a couple of years ago when I hit 8,000 miles!"

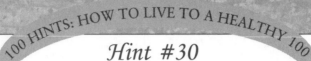

Hint #30

"Eat a vegetarian diet and keep your life simple."

Miriam Boyd
February 21, 1907
Camden, South Carolina

Miriam became a vegetarian while working as a nurse among the Hindus in India in the 1940's. And she's been one ever since. "I think it's the way we were supposed to live," she says.

Hint #31

*"Be active and be interested.
Don't withdraw from life."*

Ruth Houghton
December 30, 1911
New York, New York

Ruth was a member of a hiking club for over 35 years. She still walks 10 miles a week!

Hint #32

"Proper nutrition is vital.
Eat plenty of fruits and vegetables."

Gladys Thomas
August 6, 1911
Charlotte, Michigan

Gladys has always been a firm believer in good nutrition and maintaining a healthy body. "You've got to take care of your health," she says. "It's so easy to lose it!"

Hint #33

"Live a good, clean life with a spiritual spouse."

J. M. Gaffney
October 21, 1908
Blacksburg, South Carolina

J.M. says he's avoided smoking and drinking all his life, but attributes his longevity to a Higher Source. "I guess the good Lord just decided to let me live this long!"

Hint #34

"Drink a lot of water and get plenty of exercise."

Vester Skipper
June 5, 1913
Sylvester, Georgia

Vester says he got a lot of exercise growing up on a farm. "I've always worked hard and thought that you ought to keep moving. And I don't plan to stop now!"

Hint #35

"Take care of yourself inside and out."

Florine Taylor
December 16, 1914
Port Arthur, Texas

Florine believes it's important to maintain an attractive and healthy personal appearance to feel your very best. "I never go out of the house without my hair fixed," she smiles.

Hint #36

*"As far as health is concerned,
you reap what you sow."*

Orville MacAlpine
October 2, 1912
Bad Axe, Michigan

Orville still remembers the barn-raisings in the Scotch settlement where he grew up. "We went everywhere together as a family," he says. He and his wife, Leone, enjoy "keeping and marking accomplishments off their lists" as well as mall walking.

Hint #37

"Regular exercise is very important."

John Buchanan
June 22, 1916
Seattle, Washington

John rode his bike to work every day for eleven years, logging over 22,000 miles, and he still rides regularly. At age 80, he took a 200-mile bike ride "just for fun."

Hint #38

❖

"Stay busy and wait on yourself."

❖

Jo Brannon
November 8, 1902
Canton, North Carolina

Jo remembers years of carrying spring water into her farmhouse, and sending her four children outdoors to use the outhouse. She still keeps active, and enjoys having access to the modern "inconveniences," as she teasingly calls them.

Hint #39

"Live a clean life — no drinking or swearing."

Bertie David
June 10, 1904
Harrison, Arkansas

Bertie and her husband raised ten children on a farm near Tahlequah, Oklahoma — the capital of the Cherokee Nation. "These days I just like to relax and play bingo," she laughs.

Hint #40

"Long life is based on good, clean living."

Dr. Roy Roberts
January 20, 1898
Gilmer, Texas

Roy is one of the few remaining veterans who fought in France during World War I. After the war, he went back to school, eventually completing his PhD in agriculture. Until his retirement, he taught agriculture at the University of Arkansas.

Hint #41

"Stay away from grease!"

Herbert Hatfield
July 26, 1911
Sparta, Tennessee

Herbert, a Pontiac/Cadillac dealer for over forty years, is a strong proponent of a fat-free diet. Faced with severe heart problems in his seventies, he underwent quadruple bypass surgery. "Afterwards I completely changed the way I eat," he says, "and today the doctor says I've got a heart like a 25-year-old!"

Hint #42

"Make breakfast your biggest meal of the day."

Virginia Potter
October 20, 1909
Elkhart, Indiana

Married at 14, for over seventy years, Virginia has been making sure her family starts the day off right. "Whole grains and fresh fruit keep you strong all day!" she says. Her husband, Russell, active and alert at 93 adds, "and don't forget the buttermilk!"

Hint #43

"Eat what you want, but use good judgment."

Don Kroll
February 21, 1911
Ute, Iowa

Don enjoys remembering the pleasant times in his life. "People say you shouldn't look back, but for me it's a positive thing." Don is still active in his church, and enjoys watching sports and dabbling in the stock market.

Hint #44

"Don't work too hard, play too hard, or eat too much."

Bryce Reay
May 25, 1906
Greenfield, Ohio

Bryce is a strong supporter of "moderation in all things." He believes that moderation, "combined with my mother's prayers," is what made him the person he is today. He spends most of his time with Dollie, his bride of two years.

Hint #45

"Eat lots and lots of fresh fruit, 'an apple a day' you know!"

Jeanette Smith
May 2, 1903
Parsons, Kansas

Jeanette stays active by taking regular trips to the farmer's market. She especially loves experiencing the different tastes offered by today's exotic imports.

Hint #46

"Live life like a farm girl."

Nola Critchfield
May 28, 1903
Wellston, Oklahoma

Nola was born and raised on a farm homesteaded during the Oklahoma land rush era. She credits her long life to "good, pure farm food and lots of hard work." At age 91, she was still trimming the hedges and mowing the lawn.

Hint #47

*"Eat a little bit of everything,
but don't eat too much."*

Mollie Wallace
January 13, 1904
Oslo, Norway

Mollie moved to Montana when she was ten and has lived there ever since. She stays active by playing badminton, tennis, and bridge, and by taking friends around on little outings.

Hint #48

"Get plenty of sleep. Your body needs rest to function properly."

Magdaline Carrao
July 7, 1904
Chicago, Illinois

Magdaline taught school in Chicago for over 30 years. She still remembers her mother's lectures at the dinner table about "good and bad foods" and "balanced health habits."

Hint #49

"End your hot morning shower with cold water — the colder, the better!"

Russell L. Potter, Sr.
August 9, 1903
Aurora, Illinois

Russell owned and operated hardware stores for over half a century. In the early 1930's, he invented and built the first travel trailer he'd ever seen — complete with a toilet and hot and cold running water! "It was a real traffic stopper wherever we went!" he laughs.

Hint #50

*"Drink plenty of water each morning
and throughout the day."*

Delphia Fults
August 13, 1897
San Jose, California

Delphia drinks two eight-ounce glasses of water right after she gets up each morning. "It's kept my brain clear all these years!" she laughs.

Hint #51

"Eat lots of fresh fruit and vegetables."

Effie Jewel Church
December 2, 1898
Fannin County, Texas

Effie ("Mom" to all those who know her) raised five kids on a Texas farm, mostly on produce from the family garden. "We were too poor to buy junk food," she laughs. "Mom" still maintains a small garden, and is also a top-notch domino and Rummikub player!

Hint #52

"Do what you want to do, but don't overdo."

Josephine "Jo" Trull
February 18, 1901
Waynesville, North Carolina

Jo fondly remembers helping out at her daddy's grist mill, wading in the creek, and climbing telephone poles. "Even though those days are gone, I still believe exercise should be fun."

Hint #53

"Drink lots of fresh water, and eat right."

Auburn Roland
July 14, 1906
Burnsville, North Carolina

Auburn points out that water on the outside is good for you, too! He still remembers daily trips to the "swimmin' hole" in the river near his home. "And I still go swimming any time I get a chance!" he says.

Hint #54

*"Good food, lots of exercise —
and stay away from fast cars!"*

Nathan Rhinehart
June 1, 1906
Ellicott, New York

Nathan enjoys doing everything he can to help others. He also
loves telling stories from the "good old days" when he and his wife
ran a hunting and fishing camp in Alaska.

Hint #55

***"Don't drink or smoke,
and respect your fellow man."***

Billie Hayes Head
May 9, 1902
Aurora, Arkansas

When Billie was 19, she moved to a nearby university town to prepare for college. "It was summer and I made good money doing laundry," she remembers. That summer job blossomed into Ozark Cleaners, a huge operation she owned and operated for 42 years.

Hint #56

"Eat what you want, but don't overdo it."

Elizabeth Girtman
July 23, 1906
Woodward, Oklahoma

Elizabeth taught first graders for almost 30 years. "I really love little children," she says. Friends say you can always tell when there are children around by the big smile that lights up Elizabeth's face.

Hint #57

"A regular exercise program is vital!"

Ruth Cunningham
December 23, 1913
St. Louis, Missouri

Ruth spent years on a farm outside Kirksville, Missouri, where her husband was a professor at the university. "Living in the country, I went swimming every chance I got," Ruth says. "It's one of the best forms of exercise there is!" Today, Ruth still goes swimming several times each week.

Hint #58

"Live clean and eat right."

Genevieve Slaugh
March 7, 1906
Dry Fork, Utah

Genevieve once did social work in Iran where the people drank, bathed, and washed their clothes in the same pool. "We pointed out that they were sick a lot," she says, "and tried to get the village to install a shower." The response? "No shower," she laughs, "but they did ask for a pharmacy!"

Hint #59

"Eat the right food — carrots for the eyes, and lots of yellow vegetables!"

Florence Wear
November 2, 1897
Clarksburg, West Virginia

Although she gets "plenty of sleep," Florence is a very active senior who likes country/western music "especially for dancing"! She says until recently, a live band could get her out on the dance floor in a jiffy!

Hint #60

**"Drink a warm glass of water with
half a lemon every morning."**

Faith Ellene Potter
September 19, 1891
Aurora, Illinois

Faith spent many years teaching in one-room schoolhouses across
Indiana and Illinois. At age 100, she was still walking several miles
each week. Faith continues to read her Bible through each year —
as she has for over 40 years!

Hint #61

*"Watch what you eat,
and exercise moderately."*

Mae Richiusa
October 7, 1921
Ashland, Massachusetts

Mae, who was born without a hip, was one of the world's first hip replacement patients. She still walks regularly, enjoys swimming, and likes to dance with her husband.

Hint #62

"People who smoke are idiots!"

Lou Vabner
July 18, 1915
New York, New York

"My wife and I *were* idiots," says Lou Vabner, "and we both paid the price!" He and his wife quit smoking *many* years ago and remain fit by walking daily and playing golf.

Hint #63

*"Get aerobic exercise through
activities that interest you."*

Elenore Buchanan
November 14, 1920
Great Falls, Montana

Elenore stays active with volunteer work, providing transportation for people who are less fortunate than she. "Even if you're retired," she stresses, "you must still keep active, both mentally and physically."

Hint #64

"You need good genes, but you also have to take care of what you've got."

John Gillespie
December 18, 1919
Trenton, Tennessee

Until retirement, John worked as a pharmacist. He stays active playing with his grandkids and great-grandkids.

Hint #65

"Take a swim!"

Catherine Ewald
February 28, 1917
St. Wendel, Wisconsin

Catherine admits she's fanatical about the water, and seldom lets a day go by without swimming. "I belong to Aquafit!" she beams, "there's no better exercise than exercise in the water!"

Hint #66

*"God gave us spirit, body,
and mind — use all three!"*

Angie Grumbine
January 15, 1915
Wildomar, California

When Angie was very young, she once found her friend's mother doubled over in pain. It seems the woman liked avocados, so she'd eaten a whole pile of them! "That experience changed my entire attitude toward eating." says Angie.

Hint #67

"Stay active — both physically and socially!"

Bette Barto
August 6, 1926
Chicago, Illinois

Bette and her husband do almost everything together. She attends the health club six times a week and says she also uses the treadmill at home on a regular basis.

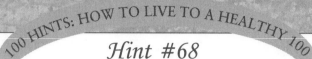

Hint #68

"Don't smoke, and have a good doctor."

Salvatore "Sam" Richiusa
December 11, 1919
South Amboy, New Jersey

Sam is a proud son of Italian immigrants. He keeps active by walking and playing golf. "I also like to dance with my wife," he says with a wink.

Hint #69

*"Whenever you're feeling
stressed, take a walk."*

Al Little
February 2, 1919
Silex, Missouri

Al stays active serving his church as a chaplain for the Los Angeles county jails. He credits his long, healthy life to an enduring faith in God.

Priorities & Outlook

Hint #70

"You don't <u>grow</u> old. You <u>get</u> old when you stop growing."

Richard Swogger
March 7, 1908
Kendallville, Indiana

Richard, a retired minister, enjoys learning from others and expressing his faith in positive ways. "Listen," he says. "You don't learn anything when you're talking!"

Hint #71

"Don't act your age!"

Vernal Augenstein
December 25, 1907
Long Point, Illinois

Vernal is admittedly "old-fashioned," she's never even worn a pair of pants! She stays active by traveling to visit friends several times a week. "Don't sit still too long!" she adds with a wink.

Hint #72

"Get up every morning believing it's going to be a nice day."

Victoria Shane
March 15, 1910
New York, New York

Though born in New York City, Victoria has spent most of her life in the West, married to a real-life cowboy. "Money's not everything," says Victoria. "Learn to do the best you can with what God gave you!"

Hint #73

"Take everything with a grain of salt."

Mildred Harris
February 19, 1911
Dewey, Oklahoma

Mildred is a "tough old gal" who believes most people "worry themselves to death." Last year she realized a lifelong dream — taking a Caribbean cruise. Her favorite part? Snorkeling in Cozumel!

Hint #74

*"Spend as much time as you
can with your family."*

Ruby Hallsted
June 19, 1914
Rudy, Arkansas

In addition to raising five children, Ruby cared for her invalid
parents for many years. She often cooked meals for her husband's
plumbing crew. Ruby still enjoys "cooking up something special"
for her children and grandchildren.

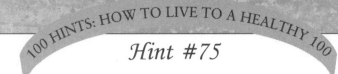

Hint #75

"Enjoy people. Spend time with your friends."

John Kozel
August 17, 1911
Brainerd, Minnesota

"Good country living" gave John a strong start in life. "It settled in my bones," he says. John makes it a point to keep in touch with his friends from college, and still enjoys spending time in the great outdoors.

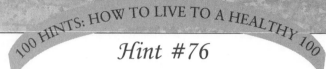

Hint #76

"Take life easy and don't waste time worrying."

Frances Gainey
July 6, 1913
Clare, Michigan

Frances taught school for many, many years. "I spent a lot of time walking," she laughs. Frances continues to stay active by walking and swimming regularly.

Hint #77

"If you plant it, take care of it."

Alice Mosby
June 12, 1909
Graysville, Tennessee

Alice says this especially applies to raising children. She also advises, "Don't dwell on the past." When her 17-year-old daughter died in 1949, she began searching to get closer to God. "And I've never stopped," she says.

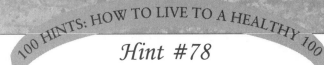

Hint #78

"Always strive to give God your best —
it's a rewarding life."

Dr. Bernard Seton
February 20, 1913
Birmingham, England

Bernard, a writer, artist, teacher, and minister, has lived in such colorful places as South Africa, Portugal, and Angola.

Hint #79

"Keep your nose out of other people's business."

Russell Woodard
April 14, 1909
Hersey, Maine

Russell grew up enjoying nature and living the life of a pioneer. "We still used oxen when I was a boy," he says. Today he brings nature inside, as he studies plants under his new microscope.

Hint #80

*"Always help those less
fortunate than yourself."*

Alice Swain
October 2, 1913
Leeton, Missouri

Alice has spent much of her life ministering to others' needs as a public health nurse. Over the years she has delivered "lots and lots of babies." She currently volunteers her time to help feed and clothe the homeless through her church's public assistance program.

Hint #81

***"Doing for others is the rent you
pay for occupying this earth."***

Ralph Smith
March 12, 1914
Waterloo, Iowa

Ralph spent much of his life as Director of Plant Services for Wesleyan colleges and universities. Today he's "the self-appointed maintenance supervisor" of the retirement center where he lives. Recently, for instance, he reworked all the down spouts so they would drain properly.

Hint #82

"Live your life caring for others."

Gladys Kenny
October 27, 1906
Mabelvale, Arkansas

Gladys made caring for others her career, meeting people's health-care needs as a nurse. Currently she enjoys sewing and crocheting, "mostly for my great-grandchildren."

Hint #83

"Just love everybody and look on the bright side."

Clara Merritt
May 2, 1908
Fort Meade, Florida

Clara has lost five sisters, four husbands, and one son, but she remains an optimistic Christian lady. "Yes, I've lost a lot, but I have a hope and a future!" she smiles.

Hint #84

"Always be completely honest —
it really is the best policy."

Carol Shafer
September 20, 1907
Spencer, Iowa

The wife of a prominent historian, Carol has known many of Washington's great intellectuals and educators. "You also should keep yourself busy," says Carol. Last year, she wrote and published a book of short stories from her life. "Mostly for the grandchildren," she says.

Hint #85

"Never give up!"

Marjorie Hobson
February 20, 1910
Cleveland, Ohio

"Life hasn't exactly been easy," says Marjorie with a sparkle in her eyes. "But I've always stuck with it!" After a difficult mid-life divorce, Marjorie supported herself for years by giving private speech lessons. One of her sons is now a writer and the other is a physics professor at a prominent university.

Hint #86

"Enjoy helping others."

Cassie Eldridge
June 10, 1911
Yale, Virginia

Cassie grew up "totin' water from the spring and washin' clothes on a washboard." Today she does laundry for her grandchildren. "I'm so thrilled to have a machine that I'm glad to do their wash!" she laughs.

Hint #87

"Don't work only for money. If you don't enjoy your job, get another one!"

Ed Hallsted
March 13, 1914
Liberty, Kentucky

Ed worked as a plumber for over 40 years, many of those in business with his sons. Over the years, Ed has also purchased, remodeled, and sold dozens of homes. He's currently working on one he calls his "playhouse."

Hint #88

❖

"Learn how to deal with your mistakes."

❖

Fisher Kenny
May 24, 1907
Trinidad, Colorado

"We all make mistakes," says Fisher, "but we don't have to keep on making the same ones!" Fisher says he's had a wonderful life, and doesn't have any regrets. His two life-long interests, woodworking and whistling, continue to provide hours of enjoyment.

Hint #89

"Treat people kindly.
Encourage those around you."

Leone MacAlpine
February 2, 1913
Caseville, Michigan

When Leone is not working in her garden, she spends her time visiting the sick, and "bringing goodies" to those who can't leave their homes.

Hint #90

"Stay single!"

Mary Russell
March 27, 1907
Cedartown, Georgia

"Most of my married friends are long gone," jokes Mary. "I think the single life agreed with me." Mary spent much of her life working as a clerk in various stores across Texas.

Hint #91

"Live life to the fullest!"

Faye Ketchersid
February 18, 1907
Gravette, Arkansas

The wife of an Arkansas farmer, Faye says she's lived a full and rewarding life. "If I had to do it over, I'd do it again!" she laughs. Faye loves to travel. She went on a bus tour of New York City when she was 80!

Hint #92

"Always be truthful with everyone."

V. C. Johnson
April 18, 1903
Montgomery County, Illinois

V.C. has been a hard-working farmer all his life. "Didn't allow much time for vacations!" he says with a wink. He adds that people who want to live a long life must make the effort to take care of themselves.

Hint #93

"Always be honest with yourself."

Viola McKee
March 25, 1900
Humboldt, Iowa

Viola spent several years teaching in a one-room schoolhouse. "There was seldom a dull moment in those days," she laughs. These days her passions are quilt-making and cats.

Hint #94

"Live your life one day at a time."

Sylvia Roddy
March 25, 1904
Paris, Arkansas

Sylvia spent many years as an operating room nurse in Arkansas and Arizona. "You never know what the future may hold," Sylvia points out, "so enjoy each day as it comes."

Hint # 95

"Live a moral and honest life."

Harriet Gibbs
April 14, 1899
Charity Shore, Pennsylvania

Harriet spent many years as a bookkeeper and secretary. She says she enjoys hard work, but her greatest love has always been reading.

Hint #96

"There's no advice to give."

Lennie Shane
December 19, 1906
Cooper County, Missouri

Though a man of few words, Lennie's active life speaks volumes. A real-life cowboy, Lennie has worked outdoors with horses and livestock all his life, "even when I didn't have to."

Hint #97

"Enjoy the act of living!"

William K. "Bill" Divers
April 12, 1905
Cincinnati, Ohio

Bill was Chairman of the Federal Home Loan Bank for two terms under President Truman, and was offered a third term under Eisenhower. "I've had an intellectually stimulating life," Divers says, "and my wife and I traveled extensively." On his 91st birthday, Bill received a hand-written note from his friend, President Bill Clinton.

Hint #98

"Working hard is good for you!"

Vina McCurdy
December 1, 1901
Gravette, Arkansas

When Vina's husband died young, leaving her with three children, family members wondered how she'd make it. "You do what you have to," says Vina with a smile. Today, she's proud of her children and grandchildren, and her over 30 years of service as an elementary school teacher and principal.

Hint #99

"Learn to see wonders that surround you."

Mary Dresbach
August 3, 1905
Van Buren, Arkansas

Since Mary's husband was a geologist, she's lived (and learned the language) in Tunisia, Ghana, "and several places you've never even heard of"! "It's been an interesting life," says Mary, "but people should remember that anywhere can be interesting if you have the right attitude."

Hint #100

*"It's not what happens to you —
it's what you do with what happens!"*

Irma Giffels
March 20, 1903
Hindsville, Arkansas

Irma says you never know where life will take you. "I still remember riding my horse to the one-room schoolhouse each day," laughs Irma. "I was only seventeen, and I was the teacher!" She later received her graduate degree in nutrition, and went on to become the director of a respected national nutrition program.

Bonus! Hint #101

"Do the right thing, even if it's difficult."

Gene Wood
September 23, 1895
Mt. Gilead, Ohio

Gene remains active, even though he lives in a retirement center. He cleans the sidewalk every day, visits with his "young girlfriend" who is 92, and occasionally quotes German poetry he learned in high school.

Bonus! Hint #102

"Conduct yourself with dignity and restraint."

Elsie Hassell
June 17, 1894
Litchfield, Nebraska

Elsie got her first paycheck as a teacher before she turned 17. "There were very few eighth grade graduates where I lived," she remembers, "so I was quite qualified for the time." After further schooling, she went on to teach high school science classes for almost 30 years.

Bonus! Hint #103

"Live a good, clean life."

Martha "Mattie" Johnson
July 7, 1891
Gravette, Arkansas

Mattie has seen a lot of changes in her lifetime. "I used to work in a store for $1.50 a day," she says, "and that was good money, too!" With 12 brothers and sisters, most of them younger, she remembers that "courting time" proved a bit difficult!

Bonus! Hint #104

"Just live it!"

Kate Haddock
February 22, 1891
Watts, Oklahoma

Kate is one of the original enrollees of the Cherokee Nation. Because of her age, relative good health, and dry sense of humor, she's often interviewed for newspaper articles or television programs.

Bonus! Hint #105

"Think young. The mind is a powerful thing."

Jack Wein
November 8, 1918
San Francisco, California

Jack is a respected representative of Secure Horizons and Senior Fit, two organizations that actively promote exercise for the elderly.

Bonus! Hint #106

"Talk to the Lord every day."

Earldean Hatch
October 27, 1906
Idabel, Oklahoma

Earldean is well-known for her young-at-heart outlook and sincere love for everyone she comes in contact with. "I don't think I've ever met a stranger," she jokes.

Bonus! Hint #107

**"Never allow yourself to get too
stressed over business."**

Gloria Ferry
March 31, 1920
Pasadena, California

Gloria is an active member of several arts foundations, and plays golf with her husband, Ray, at least twice each week. Before retiring, they were in an antique and art business together for years.

Bonus! Hint #108

"You have to have a goal in life to stay healthy."

Clarice Gillespie
July 28, 1917
Phoenix, Arizona

A lifetime homemaker, Clarice has gone from mother, to grandmother, to great-grandmother. Her final goal in life? "Just to outlive my husband, John!" she laughs.

Bonus! Hint #109

"Don't get wrapped up in extremes."

Art Grumbine
August 3, 1919
Portland, Oregon

Art says religion is the primary anchor in his life. Instead of "following the crowd," Art feels people should approach decisions by "asking yourself what God would have you do."

Bonus! Hint #110

*"When you're angry, get over it.
When you're wrong, apologize."*

Albert Rodarte
March 25, 1919
San Pedro, California

Albert was a construction worker for over 30 years, and still enjoys working with his hands. He made this comment from under a car he was working on for fun!

Bonus! Hint #111

**"Learn to trust your heavenly Father —
no matter what the future brings."**

Darrell Elder
June 16, 1912
Salina, Kansas

Darrel has seen a lot of changes in his lifetime. He still remembers riding in the wagon with his parents when his mother suddenly shouted, "Pa, grab the reins! Here comes one of them things!" "She was talking about a *car*!" laughs Darrell.

"Why, That's Nothing . . ."

Inevitably when a book like this comes out, someone will write to us and say: "Why, that's nothing! Uncle Harry just had his 109th birthday, and he still climbs Mt. Everest twice each year!"

So, here's your chance to make your older relatives and friends famous (well, sort of)! If you know an active senior who was born during or before World War I, just put together a short quote and biography like the ones in this book and send it to us! Be sure to ask their permission first, and include their phone number for verification purposes.

Who knows? They might end up in a *100 More Hints To Live To A Healthy 100!*

To mail your submissions or to write the author, address your correspondence to:

Russ L. Potter, II
c/o The Concerned Group, Inc.
P. O. Box 1000
Siloam Springs, Arkansas 72761

Russ L. Potter, II, has been interested in health and physical fitness since his early years. As a teenage member of a tumbling team whose coaches stressed a low-fat, low-sugar, vegetarian diet, he made a life-long commitment to health and fitness. At age fifty, Russ can still do handstands and 100 pushups! And, whenever possible, he plays softball and table tennis.

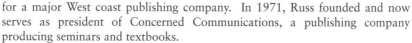

After graduating from Loma Linda University with a B.A. degree in Theology, Russ first served as a youth pastor, and then assistant sales manager and later advertising manager for a major West coast publishing company. In 1971, Russ founded and now serves as president of Concerned Communications, a publishing company producing seminars and textbooks.

Russ has been married for over thirty years to his college sweetheart, Cheryl Lee Coy. Together they have two grown children, Daniel and Angelique.

Russ says his interest in longevity "is inherited," since his aunt lived to 103 and his maternal grandfather to age 98. His father is currently 93 and his mother 87! He believes that "life is too short to even think about growing old!"

Additional copies of this book and other titles from the *100 Hints* Series are available from your local bookstore.

100 Hints: How To Stay Married For Life

Trade Life Books, Inc.
Tulsa, Oklahoma